KNOWLEDGE GUIDE TO OSTEOGENESIS IMPERFECTA

Essential Manual To Understanding The Fragile Bone Condition, Diagnosis, Treatment Options, Genetic Insights, And Living With OI

DR. AARON BRANUM

Copyright © 2024 BY DR. AARON BRANUM

All rights reserved. Except for brief quotations embodied in critical reviews and certain other noncommercial uses permitted by copyright law, no part of this publication may be reproduced, distributed, or transmitted in any form or by any means, Including photocopying, recording, or other electronic or mechanical methods, without the prior written permission of the publisher.

Disclaimer:

The data in this book, is solely meant to be informative and instructional.

This book is not intended to replace expert medical advice, diagnosis, or care. No medical, health, or other professional services are offered by the author, publisher, or any affiliated parties

Individual outcomes may differ in the practice of these therapies, which entail a variety of approaches and methodologies.

A one-on-one session with a trained or certified healthcare professional is still preferable. It is best to consult a trained healthcare provider before making any decisions regarding your health.

The author of this book is not affiliated with any specific website, product, or organization related to any of these therapies.

All reasonable measures have been taken by the author and publisher to guarantee the authenticity and dependability of the material contained in this book

Contents

CHAPTER ONE 15

KNOWING THE FUNDAMENTALS OF IMPERFECT OSTEOGENESIS 15

The Meaning And Background Of OI 15

Types And Classification Of OI 16

Genetic Factors And Heredity Arrangements 18

Fundamental Bone Biology And OI Pathophysiology 19

Important Data And Epidemiology 20

CHAPTER TWO 23

SYMPTOMS AND MEDICAL APPEARANCES ... 23

Bone Fragility And Patterns Of Fracture 24

Additional Skeletal Deviations 26

Manifestations Extra-Skeletal (Hearing, Teeth, Etc.) 27

Issues With Development And Growth 29

Impact On The Mind And Emotion 30

Diagnostic Methods 32

CHAPTER THREE 39

HEALTH CARE MANAGEMENT 39
  Synopsis Of Current Therapies 39
  Drugs (Growth Hormones, Bisphonates) 40
  Techniques For Pain Management 42
  Surgical Procedures And Their Significance 44
  Multidisciplinary Approach To Care 45
CHAPTER FOUR 49
REHABILITATION AND PHYSICAL THERAPY . 49
  Physical Therapy's Function In OI 49
  Exercise Plans And Safety Instructions 50
  Adaptive Equipment And Mobility Assistance 51
  Other Therapies And Hydrotherapy 52
  Long-Term Rehab Objectives 53
CHAPTER FIVE 55
ASPECTS RELATING TO NUTRITION 55
  Nutrition's Role In OI Management 55
  Dietary Guidelines For Maintaining Bone Health 56

Taking Care Of Nutritional Deficiencies And Weight 58

Advice For Selective Diners And Meal Organizing 58

CHAPTER SIX 61

MENTAL HEARING ASPECTS 61

Difficulties With Emotional And Mental Health 62

Coping Techniques For Families And Patients 64

Resources And Support Systems 65

Integration Of Education And Society 67

Encouraging Self-Reliance And Self-Worth 68

CHAPTER SEVEN 71

RESEARCH AND TREATMENT ADVANCES 71

Synopsis Of Ongoing Research Projects 73

Novel Therapeutics And Gene Therapy 74

Developments In Surgical Methods 75

Advances In Rehabilitation And Physical Therapy 77

Prospects For The Future And The Hope Of A Cure 78

CONCERNING THIS BOOK

"Osteogenesis Imperfecta" is a vital tool for anyone providing care, assistance, or therapy to people with this uncommon genetic condition. This extensive book sheds light on the complex features of Osteogenesis Imperfecta (OI), providing an in-depth examination of the condition's genetic foundations, clinical presentations, and the all-encompassing therapeutic strategies required to enhance patient outcomes.

The book's main focus is on offering a thorough explanation of the fundamentals of OI, along with a historical overview and a complete taxonomy of the different kinds. To emphasize the value of genetic counseling and early intervention, medical practitioners and affected families must have a thorough understanding of the genetic origins and inheritance patterns of OI. Essential insights into the fragility and distinct fracture patterns associated with OI, as well as other skeletal abnormalities and extra-skeletal manifestations like hearing loss and dental difficulties, are provided by the book's examination of bone biology and pathophysiology. These sections provide a detailed picture of the frequency and effect of OI worldwide, supplemented with important statistics and epidemiological data.

The book's meticulous approach to diagnosis is one of its strong points. It describes the significance of advanced imaging studies, the function of genetic testing, and the best practices in clinical assessment. To accurately diagnose and treat OI, a differential diagnosis must be included to identify illnesses that mimic OI. This comprehensive diagnostic approach guarantees that medical professionals can accurately diagnose OI and efficiently customize treatment plans.

Another crucial area of attention is the medical care of OI, for which the book offers a thorough summary of available therapies. It covers surgical procedures, pain management techniques, and the use of drugs such as growth hormones and bisphonates. This book's emphasis on the multidisciplinary care approach promotes teamwork in treatment plans involving multiple medical specialists to provide patients with all-encompassing care that takes their well-being into account.

The importance of physical therapy and rehabilitation in the management of OI is emphasized. The utilization of mobility aids and adapted equipment, safe exercise regimens, and the importance of physical therapy are all covered in the book. These useful recommendations aid patients in preserving their mobility and enhancing their quality of life. The advantages of hydrotherapy and long-term rehabilitation objectives are also spelled out, offering a road map for maintaining physical health.

A section on dietary guidelines, necessary supplements, and addressing nutritional deficits gives adequate regard to nutritional issues. For OI sufferers to maintain their general health and bone health, this knowledge is essential. Families and caregivers may find the practical advice on meal planning and handling dietary problems especially helpful.

OI's psychosocial components are thoughtfully and empathetically discussed. The book examines the difficulties with emotional and mental health that patients and their families encounter, providing coping mechanisms and emphasizing the value of support networks. It emphasizes the value of social and educational integration, which helps people with OI become more independent and confident in themselves.

This book covers fascinating new ground in research and treatment. With discussions of new developments in surgery and physical therapy, gene therapy prospects, and ongoing research projects, there is optimism for future discoveries and possible treatments.

It is imperative to have an informed viewpoint regarding the constantly changing field of occupational injury treatment and care.

Carefully considered answers to frequently asked questions are offered to address typical issues and offer helpful guidance on handling OI.

The value of the book as a go-to resource for patients, families, and healthcare professionals is increased by this part.

All things considered, "Osteogenesis Imperfecta" is an invaluable resource that provides readers with thorough, current information that gives them hope and knowledge for improved management and treatment of this difficult condition.

14

CHAPTER ONE

KNOWING THE FUNDAMENTALS OF IMPERFECT OSTEOGENESIS

The Meaning And Background Of OI

Osteogenesis Imperfecta (OI) is a hereditary illness characterized by brittle bone disease and fragile, easily broken bones, frequently with little or no obvious reason.

The disease is caused by a malfunction in the synthesis of collagen, which is an essential structural protein in bone tissue.

Ancient records exist regarding OI, and the first thorough medical description appeared in the 19th century.

Advances in molecular biology and genetic study have led to a deeper knowledge of the illness than was initially known.

Types And Classification Of OI

Based on genetic variations and the intensity of symptoms, OI is categorized into multiple kinds.

Four main categories are identified by the Sillence categorization system, which was developed in 1979. Other forms have been identified more since.

Type I: The most frequent and moderate variant, with blue sclerae (a bluish tint to the whites of the eyes), slight bone deformities, and easily fractured bones. Adulthood may bring on hearing loss.

Type II: significant variant that is frequently fatal soon after birth as a result of respiratory issues brought on by underdeveloped lungs and significant bone abnormalities.

Type III: Similarly severe, with a notable skeletal malformation that either develops in early childhood or is present from birth. Some people may be small in stature and rely heavily on wheelchairs.

Type IV: A slight to moderate bone malformation, readily fractured bones, and normal sclerae are characteristics of this intermediate variant. Patients frequently vary in height and may or may not utilize assistive technology.

With the identification of kinds V through XI more recently, each with distinct genetic and clinical characteristics, the diversity of OI has been better understood.

Genetic Factors And Heredity Arrangements

Type I collagen is encoded by the COL1A1 and COL1A2 genes, and mutations in these genes are the main cause of OI.

These mutations decrease bone structure by interfering with collagen's normal synthesis, structure, and function.

The majority of OI types have autosomal dominant inheritance, which means that the disorder can be caused by a single mutated copy of the gene in each cell. Certain uncommon variants, on the other hand, are inherited in an autosomal recessive fashion, meaning that each cell must have two different copies of the gene.

Most cases of OI are caused by spontaneous mutations, in which the condition has no family history. For families affected by OI, genetic testing and counseling are essential because they help with early diagnosis and care and provide information on the likelihood of transferring the disorder to kids.

Fundamental Bone Biology And OI Pathophysiology

The dynamic structures known as bones are made up of minerals like calcium phosphate and a collagen matrix. Defective collagen in OI leads to a weakened bone matrix, which makes bones brittle and more prone to breaking.

Abnormal bone architecture results from disruptions in the normal process of bone remodeling, which involves the resorption of bone by osteoclasts and the production of new bone by osteoblasts.

In addition to skeletal fragility, anomalies in connective tissues across the body are also part of the pathophysiology of OI. In addition to fractures, this can cause hypermobility in the joints, easily bruised skin, and dental problems because of poor dentin quality.

Important Data And Epidemiology

With an estimated prevalence of 1 in 15,000 to 20,000 births, OI is a rare illness. Depending on the demographic and the particular kind of OI, the incidence and severity can differ significantly.

Type I is the most common, making up around half of all instances, although Type II is uncommon and is usually detected at birth because of how severe it is.

Even though it is uncommon, OI affects people all over the world, with no discernible racial or ethnic distinctions in its prevalence. Many people with OI now have a better outlook thanks to advancements in genetic research and medical care, which allows for improved symptom control and a higher quality of life.

However, OI continues to be a chronic illness that necessitates extensive and interdisciplinary approaches to treatment to manage its various clinical symptoms.

CHAPTER TWO

SYMPTOMS AND MEDICAL APPEARANCES

Individual differences in severity are observed in the range of symptoms and clinical manifestations associated with Osteogenesis Imperfecta (OI). Bone fragility, which frequently fractures even with little damage, is one of the main signs. Prenatal ultrasounds can reveal multiple fractures or bowing of the long bones in babies with severe types of OI, which can occur even before birth.

In addition to fractures, skeletal abnormalities including bone malformations, short height, and joint laxity can be seen in patients with OI. These anomalies may impair movement and make it harder to carry out daily tasks. Due to sclera thinness, some people may also develop blue sclerae, which is a bluish tint to the whites of the eyes.

OI can also have an impact on the respiratory system, which can result in respiratory issues including pneumonia or respiratory distress. This is especially prevalent in those who have severe variations of the illness. Another extra-skeletal symptom of OI that some people experience is hearing loss, which can range in severity and necessitate treatment with devices like hearing aids.

Bone Fragility And Patterns Of Fracture

Bone fragility, which predisposes people to fractures with little damage or even without any apparent reason, is the defining feature of Osteogenesis Imperfecta (OI).

OI patients have brittle, easily broken bones because of structural or collagen synthesis abnormalities.

Depending on the nature and severity of the illness, OI can have a variety of fracture patterns. In less severe kinds, fractures can happen less frequently and might only happen in particular places, like the long bones in the arms and legs. On the other hand, in more serious cases, fractures involving numerous bones may occur on their own or as a result of normal actions like lifting or carrying goods.

Furthermore, fractures can range in severity from minor to severe, with some resulting in very little pain and others causing severe pain and functional impairment. Because of the underlying bone fragility in people with OI, fractures may also mend more slowly in these individuals. Careful management and rehabilitation are necessary to avoid complications like malunion or nonunion.

Additional Skeletal Deviations

People with Osteogenesis Imperfecta (OI) may have a variety of skeletal abnormalities that can impair their mobility and general function, in addition to bone fragility and fractures. Bone deformities like scoliosis, or abnormal curvature of the spine, or improper formation of the pelvis or ribs, might be among these anomalies.

Additionally, people with OI may be short in stature, which can be caused by a variety of conditions such as delayed growth, skeletal anomalies, or compression fractures of the spine. A person's self-esteem may be affected by short stature, and treatments like growth hormone therapy or orthopedic surgery may be necessary to increase height and general function.

Another common skeletal anomaly observed in people with OI is joint laxity, which is defined as increased joint flexibility or looseness. Laxity in the joints can lead to instability and raise the possibility of recurring injuries or dislocations. For people with OI, bracing and physical therapy may be suggested to help stabilize the joints and increase mobility.

Manifestations Extra-Skeletal (Hearing, Teeth, Etc.)

Osteogenesis Imperfecta (OI) can cause extra-skeletal symptoms in addition to skeletal problems by affecting multiple other systems in the body.

Hearing loss is a typical extra-skeletal manifestation that can result from harm to the inner ear structures or anomalies in the creation of the middle ear bones.

In addition, dental anomalies including tooth discoloration, enamel flaws, or heightened cavity susceptibility may be experienced by those who have OI. Oral health may be impacted by several dental problems, which may need ongoing dental care as well as procedures like orthodontics or dental restorations.

Furthermore, respiratory issues such as asthma or restrictive lung disease, which can impair breathing and respiratory function, may be present in people with OI. To avoid problems and enhance the quality of life for those suffering from OI, it is imperative to conduct routine monitoring and management of respiratory symptoms.

Issues With Development And Growth

Concerns about growth and development are frequent among people with Osteogenesis Imperfecta (OI), especially in younger patients. In comparison to their classmates, children with OI may face delays in growth and development due to skeletal abnormalities and bone fragility.

A child's capacity to engage in physical activities might be impacted by conditions including persistent discomfort, recurrent fractures, or limited mobility, which can also affect the child's general growth and development. Children with OI can benefit from early intervention in the form of physical therapy, occupational therapy, and nutritional support to maximize their growth and development.

Furthermore, some OI patients may experience delayed puberty, which can further impede growth and development. When delayed puberty is a concern, hormonal medication or methods to promote puberty may be taken into consideration. To guarantee the best results, healthcare professionals must keep a careful eye on the growth and development of patients with OI and respond quickly to any concerns.

Impact On The Mind And Emotion

The psychological and emotional effects of having osteogenesis imperfecta (OI) can be profound for both the affected person and their family. Feelings of irritation, worry, or despair might result from managing physical restrictions, frequent fractures, and chronic pain.

Furthermore, issues related to social acceptance, self-worth, and body image can surface, especially in adolescence and early adulthood. Due to their physical peculiarities, people with OI may have difficulties in social interactions, as well as bullying or prejudice.

Moreover, worry, remorse, or feelings of inadequacy can be experienced by family members and caregivers of people with OI when providing care for a loved one with complicated medical needs. Access to comprehensive support services, including peer support groups, mental health counseling, and community resources, is crucial for people with OI and their families to address the psychological and emotional effects of living with OI and to foster resilience and overall well-being.

Diagnostic Methods

Healthcare practitioners use a multifaceted strategy to appropriately analyze Osteogenesis Imperfecta (OI) to diagnose it. A complete history taking and extensive clinical assessment usually precede the process. This includes reviewing the patient's past medical records, family history, and any OI-related symptoms or indicators.

Finding the distinctive characteristics of OI, such as bone fragility, deformities, and fracture susceptibility, depends heavily on clinical assessment.

Another essential step in the diagnosis procedure is genetic testing. Geneticists can find mutations in OI-associated genes like COL1A1 and COL1A2 by examining the patient's DNA. This aids in the diagnosis confirmation and offers important details regarding the particular subtype of OI that the patient has. To help patients and their families comprehend the consequences of the diagnosis and make educated decisions regarding treatment and future planning, genetic counseling is frequently offered in addition to testing.

Imaging investigations are an essential part of the diagnosis process for OI, in addition to clinical evaluation and genetic testing. To evaluate the structure, density, and presence of any anomalies in the bone, X-rays, CT scans, and MRI scans are frequently utilized. By visualizing fractures, skeletal abnormalities, and other distinctive characteristics of OI, these imaging modalities help medical professionals diagnose and plan treatments.

Assessments of bone density and quality are also crucial diagnostic instruments for evaluating organ injury. Bone mineral density and general bone health are commonly evaluated by Dual-energy X-ray absorptiometry (DEXA) scans. OI patients may have far lower bone density than typical, which raises their risk of fracture. Healthcare providers can more accurately assess the severity of a patient's ailment and adjust treatment plans by measuring bone density and quality.

Differential Diagnosis: OI-Mimicking Conditions

Even though Osteogenesis Imperfecta (OI) has unique clinical characteristics, it can occasionally be difficult to distinguish it from other illnesses that exhibit comparable symptoms. Numerous conditions might resemble OI, which could cause confusion or incorrect diagnoses during the diagnostic procedure. To arrive at an appropriate diagnosis, healthcare providers must take into account these differential diagnoses and do comprehensive evaluations.

Osteoporosis, a disorder marked by decreasing bone density and increased fracture risk, is one condition that mimics OI. Osteoporosis patients may have skeletal abnormalities and frequent fractures, similar to OI patients. On the other hand, osteoporosis usually develops later in life and is more frequently linked to age and hormonal fluctuations. It is frequently necessary to carefully evaluate clinical symptoms, genetic testing, and imaging examinations to distinguish between osteoporosis and osteopenia.

Hypophosphatasia, a hereditary illness affecting bone mineralization, is another condition to take into account in the differential diagnosis of OI. People who have hypophosphatasia could exhibit skeletal deformities and fractures that are comparable to those who have OI. On the other hand, mutations in the ALPL gene, which codes for tissue-neutralizing alkaline phosphatase, result in hypophosphatasia. By determining the underlying genetic issue, genetic testing can assist in differentiating between hypophosphatasia and OI.

Furthermore, the signs of osteomalacia and rickets, two metabolic bone disorders, may overlap with those of OI. These disorders can cause fractures and deformities in the bones because they are caused by irregularities in the metabolism of minerals. Differential diagnosis can be facilitated by the unique biochemical anomalies that normally distinguish them. Differentiating between OI and metabolic bone disorders requires laboratory testing, imaging studies, and clinical assessment.

In conclusion, despite having distinct clinical and genetic characteristics, osteogenesis imperfecta (OI) is similar to several other disorders. Accurately diagnosing OI and distinguishing it from other conditions with similar presentations requires a comprehensive diagnostic evaluation that takes into account differential diagnoses, genetic testing, imaging investigations, and clinical assessment. Healthcare professionals may guarantee prompt and correct diagnosis, which will result in suitable management and treatment methods, by thoroughly assessing every facet of the patient's medical history and carrying out the necessary tests.

CHAPTER THREE

HEALTH CARE MANAGEMENT

Synopsis Of Current Therapies

An all-encompassing medical approach is necessary for the management of Osteogenesis Imperfecta (OI). Patients and their families must comprehend the latest treatments that are available. The goals of these therapies are to increase bone density, lessen the risk of fractures, control pain, and improve quality of life overall.

Medications are a major component of the treatments used today. For example, doctors frequently prescribe bisphosphonates to patients to boost bone density and lower their risk of fracture. By preventing bone resorption, these medications strengthen bones. Research is still being done to determine the best dosages and long-term effects of these substances.

Growth Hormone (GH) is another drug utilized in the treatment of OI. The goal of GH treatment for kids with OI is to increase their growth and bone mineral density. Growth hormone (GH) can assist improve skeletal strength and lower the risk of fracture by promoting bone creation and growth. Close observation is required, though, as individual differences may exist in its efficacy.

Drugs (Growth Hormones, Bisphonates)

Patients with OI are frequently offered a class of medications called bisphosphonates, which enhance bone density and lower the risk of fracture.

These drugs function by preventing the resorption of bone, hence promoting bone strength. Depending on the patient's age and the severity of their ailment, they are usually given intravenously or orally.

GH therapy is an additional treatment option available to people with OI, especially youngsters.

By promoting bone development and growth, GH lowers the risk of fracture and increases bone mineral density.

This therapy needs to be closely monitored to determine its efficacy and modify dosage, as it is frequently used in conjunction with other therapies.

It's crucial to remember that while GH treatment and bisphosphonates have both demonstrated potential in treating OI symptoms, they might not be appropriate for everyone.

Before starting any drug regimen, it is important to take into account the age, medical history, and general condition of each patient. Healthcare experts also need to keep a tight eye on long-term results and possible negative effects.

Techniques For Pain Management

Treatment for OI must include pain management since people with this illness frequently have chronic pain as a result of fractures and bone abnormalities.

For OI patients, a variety of techniques are used to reduce pain and enhance quality of life.

Pain management and increased mobility can be achieved with non-pharmacological methods such as physical therapy, occupational therapy, and assistive technology.

By strengthening muscles, promoting joint function, and increasing general physical function, these therapies lessen the load on brittle bones.

For OI patients, pharmaceutical treatments are available for pain management in addition to non-pharmacological approaches.

NSAIDs, or nonsteroidal anti-inflammatory medicines, are frequently used to treat musculoskeletal conditions such as fractures by reducing pain and inflammation.

NSAIDs should be used with caution, though, as they raise the possibility of gastrointestinal bleeding and other side effects.

Surgical Procedures And Their Significance

In severe cases or with consequences including spinal abnormalities and recurring fractures, surgical procedures are essential to the therapy of OI.

The goals of these operations are to enhance overall bone function and quality of life, stabilize fractures, and treat abnormalities.

Intramedullary rodding, a typical surgical procedure for osteogenesis imperfecta (OI), involves inserting metal rods into the long bones to give support and avoid fractures.

Children who have severe bone abnormalities or recurring fractures that severely limit their mobility and quality of life are frequently candidates for this therapy.

Additional surgical procedures could involve joint replacements to increase the range of motion and lessen pain, spinal fusion to stabilize the spine, and corrective osteotomies to realign bones.

The decision to have surgery is based on several variables, including the patient's goals and preferences, the location of fractures or deformities, and the severity of the ailment.

Multidisciplinary Approach To Care

To effectively manage OI and meet the varied needs of patients, a multidisciplinary treatment strategy is necessary.

Healthcare professionals from several areas, such as orthopedics, genetics, physical therapy, occupational therapy, and pain management, collaborate in this strategy.

In the multidisciplinary treatment team, orthopedic specialists are essential because they have the knowledge and experience to handle skeletal abnormalities, fractures, and other OI-related problems.

In addition to offering advice on family planning and genetic testing, genetic counselors assist families in understanding the underlying genetic causes of OI.

Occupational therapists and physical therapists use targeted exercises, assistive technology, and adaptive techniques to help patients gain more strength, mobility, and functional independence.

Pain management professionals create individualized treatment programs to help people with OI manage chronic pain and enhance their quality of life.

A multidisciplinary care strategy makes sure that patients with OI receive complete and all-encompassing treatment by combining several healthcare professions and services.

This method takes into account the patient's long-term health and quality of life in addition to their acute medical demands.

To maximize results and deliver patient-centered care, team members must effectively coordinate and communicate with one another.

CHAPTER FOUR

REHABILITATION AND PHYSICAL THERAPY

Physical Therapy's Function In OI

Physical therapy is essential for managing Osteogenesis Imperfecta (OI) since it reduces the risk of fractures and deformities while enhancing function, strength, and mobility. Physical therapy's main objective is to improve OI patients' quality of life by attending to their unique demands and difficulties.

Physical therapists customize treatment regimens for each patient based on their condition, taking into account things like weak muscles, flexible joints, and fragile bones. Throughout the rehabilitation process, they make use of a variety of techniques and modalities to enhance muscle strength, balance, and range of motion while maintaining patient safety.

Exercise Plans And Safety Instructions

Exercise regimens tailored for people with OI are made to reduce the risk of fractures while enhancing bone health, muscle strength, and general physical fitness. These workout regimens usually combine resistance training, aerobic exercises, and weight-bearing exercises.

To avoid injuries, safety precautions are crucial in exercise regimens for people with OI. Patients are taught safe movement practices, correct body mechanics, and ways to prevent fractures from high-impact activities by physical therapists.

By each patient's capacities and tolerance levels, they also offer advice on the proper escalation and intensity of exercise.

Adaptive Equipment And Mobility Assistance

For people with OI, mobility assistance and adaptive equipment are essential for improving their independence and safety.

To maximize functional mobility, physical therapists evaluate each patient's needs for mobility and recommend the right assistive equipment, such as walkers, wheelchairs, or orthotic devices.

Adaptive equipment can make daily living activities more comfortable and productive for people with OI while also lowering their risk of injury.

Examples of this equipment include customized seating arrangements and assistive gadgets. To guarantee appropriate fitting and technique, physical therapists offer instruction and direction on the use of these aids.

Other Therapies And Hydrotherapy

For people with OI, hydrotherapy, also referred to as aquatic therapy, is a useful addition to conventional physical therapy.

Water's buoyancy provides resistance for cardiovascular training and muscle strengthening while lessening the burden on brittle bones. In a secure and encouraging setting, hydrotherapy can enhance the range of motion, flexibility, and general physical function.

Apart from hydrotherapy, the rehabilitation program may involve additional therapeutic modalities like electrical stimulation, manual therapy, and ultrasound to target particular OI symptoms and demands.

The purpose of physical therapy interventions is to maximize functional results and quality of life for each patient, taking into account their unique condition and reaction to treatment.

Long-Term Rehab Objectives

For those with OI, the main objectives of long-term rehabilitation are to maximize physical function, reduce comorbidities, and improve general well-being throughout a lifetime. Physical therapists collaborate with patients, families, and other medical professionals to create meaningful goals that are achievable and take into account each person's unique requirements and priorities.

Increasing mobility and independence, lowering pain and discomfort, avoiding fractures and deformities, and encouraging engagement in fulfilling activities and social interactions are a few examples of these objectives.

Physical therapists enable people with OI to reach their maximum potential and enjoy life to the fullest despite the obstacles presented by their condition through continuous examination, education, and support.

CHAPTER FIVE

ASPECTS RELATING TO NUTRITION

Osteogenesis Imperfecta (OI) is a hereditary condition characterized by brittle bones, for which nutrition is essential to management.

In those with OI, a healthy diet can promote bone health, reduce the risk of fractures, and improve general well-being.

Comprehending the importance of nutrition and putting suitable food plans into practice are crucial elements of managing occupational illness.

Nutrition's Role In OI Management

For those with OI, nutrition is essential since it directly affects bone density and strength. To promote bone production and reduce the risk of fractures, an adequate intake of important nutrients such as calcium, vitamin D, protein, and other micronutrients is required. Maintaining optimum nutrition becomes even more important to offset the impact of OI on skeletal health, as persons with the disorder already have frail bones.

Dietary Guidelines For Maintaining Bone Health

It's critical to concentrate on a balanced diet full of nutrients that support bone growth and strength to promote bone health in people with OI.

To promote bone mineralization, a diet rich in calcium-rich foods such as dairy products, leafy greens, and fortified meals should be consumed.

Similarly, calcium absorption and bone metabolism depend on vitamin D-rich meals like fatty fish, egg yolks, and fortified cereals.

Vitamin D, calcium, and other supplements

For those with OI, supplements may be required in addition to food sources to guarantee sufficient consumption of particular nutrients.

While vitamin D supplements help with calcium absorption and use, calcium supplements can help meet daily requirements for bone mineralization.

It's critical to speak with medical professionals to identify the right supplement dosage based on each person's needs and the degree of their inflammatory response.

Taking Care Of Nutritional Deficiencies And Weight

For those with OI, maintaining a healthy weight is crucial to supporting overall bone health and lowering their risk of fractures.

However, because of things like diminished mobility or weaker muscles, it can be difficult to reach and stay at a healthy weight.

Eating a healthy diet and engaging in regular exercise based on one's ability can help control weight and avoid the nutritional deficits that are frequently linked to autoimmune illness.

Advice For Selective Diners And Meal Organizing

Meal planning and inventive food selections can significantly improve the quality of life for people with OI who may have trouble eating or who follow particular diets.

Ensuring proper nutrition can be facilitated by incorporating foods that are high in nutrients and both palatable and simple to eat.

You may educate finicky eaters to appreciate a varied and well-balanced diet by experimenting with different textures, flavors, and presentation techniques.

Involving people in meal preparation and planning also gives them the power to choose healthier foods and form wholesome eating habits.

CHAPTER SIX

MENTAL HEARING ASPECTS

Osteogenesis Imperfecta (OI) can cause patients and their families to face a variety of psychological difficulties. Handling these factors is essential for overall quality of life, from maintaining mental well-being to adjusting to physical restrictions.

The effect on identity and self-image is one important factor. Because of their physical characteristics, people with OI may encounter misconceptions or preconceptions from society. Feelings of uneasiness or poor self-esteem may result from this.

Consequently, it is crucial to promote a good self-image and develop resilience despite criticism from others. Promoting open communication and offering assistance can aid in the development of a strong sense of self-worth in people.

Furthermore, negotiating social interactions might be difficult. Peers might not fully comprehend the illness, which could make you feel excluded or alone.

Meaningful relationships and friendships can be facilitated by educating others about OI and encouraging inclusivity.

Fighting social obstacles requires fostering supportive situations where people feel appreciated and accepted for who they are.

Difficulties With Emotional And Mental Health

The psychological and mental health difficulties linked to OI can differ greatly from person to person. Some may struggle to adjust to frequent medical treatments or deal with uncertainty about the future, while others may experience anxiety or sadness associated with their disease.

Taking care of chronic pain is one prevalent problem. OI can result in acute pain episodes or chronic discomfort that interferes with day-to-day activities and emotional health.

Reducing suffering and enhancing general quality of life need the application of efficient pain management approaches, such as medicine, physical therapy, or relaxation methods.

Managing fractures and their aftermath is another important topic. OI patients frequently suffer fractures, which call for medical attention and rehabilitation.

Fractures can cause both physical and psychological discomfort, which can be detrimental to one's mental health. Providing all-encompassing assistance, such as peer support groups, emotional counseling, and access to medical treatment, can help people develop resilience and cope with life's obstacles.

Coping Techniques For Families And Patients

People with OI and their families need to have efficient coping mechanisms to manage the difficulties posed by the illness. Promoting a sense of empowerment and control is one strategy.

Activating people to speak up for their needs and take an active role in decisions about their care can boost their sense of self-efficacy and autonomy.

Furthermore, encouraging flexible coping strategies can assist people in skillfully handling stress and ambiguity. This could include doing mindfulness exercises, using relaxation methods, or asking friends and medical experts for social support. Coping and resilience can also be facilitated by fostering open communication within the family and by establishing a safe space where emotions are accepted.

Resources And Support Systems

To effectively navigate the complexities of their disease, people with OI and their families must have access to support networks and resources.

Orthopedic surgeons, genetic counselors, and physical therapists are examples of medical specialists who specialize in OI and can offer individualized care and assistance.

When it comes to bringing people together through similar experiences and offering emotional support, peer support groups and online communities are also quite helpful. These platforms facilitate the exchange of guidance, information, and coping mechanisms among users, so promoting a feeling of community and comprehension.

Additionally, families and people can be empowered to become knowledgeable advocates for their community and themselves by having access to advocacy organizations and educational resources.

These sites offer insightful knowledge about OI management, available treatments, and individual rights, empowering users to take charge of their health and seek out the assistance they require.

Integration Of Education And Society

For people with OI to succeed academically and socially, it is imperative to support their educational and social integration.

This could entail working together with educators and school administrators to put in place modifications that take care of physical needs and encourage diversity in the classroom.

Fostering acceptance and support among peers can also be achieved through promoting peer education and understanding of OI.

Giving people with OI the chance to take part in extracurricular activities and social gatherings might help them become more confident and socialized.

Furthermore, using technology and online learning environments can make education more accessible for those with OI who would find it difficult to attend traditional educational settings because of mobility issues or health issues.

All students can benefit from flexible and customized support offered by virtual learning environments, which guarantee equal access to educational possibilities.

Encouraging Self-Reliance And Self-Worth

Encouraging self-reliance and self-worth is essential for people with OI to grow resilient and prosper despite their physical limitations. This could entail encouraging people to participate actively in their everyday activities and self-care regimens and putting an emphasis on their strengths rather than their weaknesses.

Developing a sense of independence in making decisions and addressing problems can improve a person's competence and confidence. Giving people the chance to develop their skills and set goals, through volunteer work or career training, for example, can help them feel more accomplished and purposeful.

Building a network of mentors, family members, and friends who believe in a person's potential and ability is also crucial for developing resilience and self-worth. No matter how minor, celebrating successes and milestones helps one maintain a positive self-image and spurs further progress.

CHAPTER SEVEN

RESEARCH AND TREATMENT ADVANCES

Osteogenesis Imperfecta (OI) sufferers now have hope and promise thanks to major advancements in the disease's study and therapy in recent years. To enhance patients' quality of life and ultimately discover a solution, scientists and medical professionals from all over the world have committed themselves to deciphering the complexity of OI.

One important development is our growing knowledge of the genetic causes of OI. The development of sophisticated genomic technology has allowed scientists to identify a large number of genes linked to osteogenesis imperfecta (OI), providing insight into the complex processes that underlie the creation and upkeep of bones. This increased knowledge opens the door to more specialized treatments and therapies based on the unique genetic profiles of individual patients.

The creation of innovative treatments and gene therapy represents another fascinating area of OI research. By fixing the genetic abnormalities causing the illness, gene therapy has enormous promise to treat OI from its core cause. Although gene therapy is still in its experimental stages, preclinical studies have yielded encouraging results, providing promise for future advancements in the treatment of OI.

In addition, scientists are investigating novel biologics and pharmaceuticals that have the potential to strengthen bones and lower the risk of fracture in people with osteoporosis.

Synopsis Of Ongoing Research Projects

Research efforts in OI are currently spanning many different fields, from biomechanics to molecular genetics, which reflects the multidisciplinary approach required to address this complicated condition thoroughly.

The advancement of OI research has been fueled by the cooperative efforts of scientists, physicians, and patient advocacy groups, creating a lively and dynamic research community committed to bettering patient outcomes.

A primary goal of current research endeavors is to clarify the molecular pathways that underlie the pathophysiology of OI.

Through disentangling the complex interactions among genetic mutations, collagen synthesis, and bone metabolism, scientists hope to identify new targets for therapeutic intervention and create more potent approaches to treating osteoporosis. Researchers can now see bone composition and structure in unprecedented detail because of advanced imaging techniques like MRI and micro-CT scanning. This information is crucial for understanding how diseases proceed and how treatments work.

Novel Therapeutics And Gene Therapy

With the potential to address the underlying genetic abnormalities causing the condition, gene therapy offers great promise as a potential treatment for OI.

Gene therapy works by inserting functional copies of the damaged genes into the target cells, which restores normal cellular function and lessens the symptoms of the disease. Gene therapy for OI is still in the early stages, but preclinical research has produced promising results that are opening the door to human clinical trials.

Researchers are looking into new biologics and pharmaceuticals in addition to gene therapy to strengthen bones and lower the risk of fracture in people with OI. For instance, bisphosphonates are frequently used to treat OI patients to improve bone density and lower the risk of fracture. However new treatments like anti-sclerostin antibodies and sclerostin inhibitors provide fresh ways to help OI patients' fracture resistance and bone quality.

Developments In Surgical Methods

In the treatment of OI, surgery is essential, especially when there are severe skeletal abnormalities or repeated fractures.

The treatment of OI has completely changed as a result of recent advancements in surgical procedures, which reduce surgical risks and consequences and enable more accurate and efficient correction of skeletal defects.

The use of intramedullary rodding procedures to stabilize lengthy bones in individuals with OI is one noteworthy accomplishment.

Surgically inserted into the medullary canal of damaged bones, intramedullary rods made of titanium or stainless steel offer structural support and guard against fractures.

Compared to conventional external fixation techniques, this minimally invasive technology promotes shorter recovery times and lowers the risk of postoperative problems.

Advances In Rehabilitation And Physical Therapy

For people with OI, physical therapy and rehabilitation are essential to optimizing function and mobility. The way OI patients are treated has changed dramatically as a result of recent advancements in physical therapy methods and rehabilitation strategies, allowing them to enjoy more independent and active lives.

Using water therapy for people with OI is one cutting-edge strategy. Aquatic treatment leverages the buoyancy of water to decrease the stress on delicate bones while allowing for modest resistance workouts and range of motion activities. Without placing unnecessary strain on the skeletal system, this low-impact exercise helps increase cardiovascular fitness, joint flexibility, and muscle strength.

Prospects For The Future And The Hope Of A Cure

For those who are living with OI, the future is bright because research is still being done to expand scientific understanding and innovation. Although there is still no known cure for OI, new developments in pharmacology, surgery, and gene therapy provide hope for more effective therapies and better patient outcomes.

One of the main objectives going forward is the creation of more individualized and precision-based OI medicines. Researchers want to optimize therapy efficacy and minimize negative effects by customizing treatment approaches to each patient's unique genetic composition by utilizing advances in genomic medicine and molecular biology.

Apart from the progress in therapeutic interventions, there are also endeavors to improve the quality of life and supportive care provided to individuals with OI. To increase awareness, advance research, and fight for improved access to healthcare services for OI patients and their families, patient advocacy groups and support networks are essential.

Overall, even if there are still obstacles to overcome, the combined efforts of the scientific community, medical professionals, and patient advocates provide those who live with OI hope for a better future. We may work toward the ultimate objective of bettering outcomes and discovering a treatment for this uncommon genetic condition with sustained focus and perseverance.

www.ingramcontent.com/pod-product-compliance
Lightning Source LLC
Chambersburg PA
CBHW071841210526
45479CB00001B/234